Confessions of a
TERMINATOR
PHYSICIAN'S PERSPECTIVE FROM THE OTHER SIDE

E. K Otah, MD

Gotham Books

30 N Gould St.
Ste. 20820, Sheridan, WY 82801
https://gothambooksinc.com/

Phone: 1 (307) 464-7800

© 2024 E. K Otah, MD. All rights reserved.

No part of this book may be reproduced, stored in a retrieval system, or transmitted by any means without the written permission of the author.

Published by Gotham Books (May 21, 2025)

ISBN: 979-8-3482-6919-7 (H)
ISBN: 979-8-3482-6917-3 (P)
ISBN: 979-8-3482-6918-0 (E)

Because of the dynamic nature of the Internet, any web addresses or links contained in this book may have changed since publication and may no longer be valid.

The views expressed in this work are solely those of the author and do not necessarily reflect the views of the publisher, and the publisher hereby disclaims any responsibility for them.

TABLE OF CONTENTS

FOREWORD iv
PREFACE vi
INTRODUCTION ix
JUNIOR, INTERMEDIATE AND SENIOR ROTATIONS. 1
    The New Life; The actual beginning 5
    The medical college years 8
    A fish out of water 12
FIRST BLOOD 15
THE MUNDANE 20
THE CHALLENGE 26
    The beginning of beginnings 28
    The turnabout 30
THE EXODUS 35
THE RECKONING 39
THE REAPER COMETH 43
LESSONS FROM CONFESSIONS 52

FOREWORD

I want to appreciate Dr. Ken Otah for writing this wonderful book "Confessions of A Terminator".

Not only did it make for an exciting read but it is also packed with the power of transformation for anyone who reads and understands the contents.

If this was a fictional material it would have been very impactful, so, the fact that it relays true accounts makes it not only impactful but a tool for the impartation of God's grace of forgiveness and deliverance to everyone that comes to Him.

This book, "Confessions of A Terminator", showcases the depravity of man without God. God spoke about how fallen man's heart/imagination is desperately wicked. This book, makes it so easy for one to understand the real state of fallen man, and man's need for the redemptive work of Jesus Christ.

More than a memoir, I see this as a strong evangelistic tool, as it easily displays mankind's need of a Saviour because of our state of spiritual death following the fall.

One of the most impressive things about this book is how it portrays God as one who is ever merciful. It also fully displays the transforming power of His unfailing and unconditional love for fallen man.

I am also intrigued that this book not only brings readers who are not saved to a point of decision where they must choose or reject Jesus Christ, but it also helps the saved reader to embrace a life that brings honor and glory to God. Another key thing that stands out as I read through the manuscript is the need for true discipleship. Salvation is not just about leading someone in saying the "sinner's prayer" but involves guiding that individual to follow a path that ensures that they bear fruit worthy of repentance. Once again, I thank Dr. Ken Otah for being so transparent with his own life, in writing this, so that readers can truly embrace the transforming power of God's grace.

Dr. David Ibeleme
Bishop & President Victorious Outreach Faith Ministries World
Trinidad & Tobago

PREFACE

Re Foundations and Confessions: A Requiem

This book is dedicated to the numerous lives, gifts from the creator that have been returned back to the giver. Over time there have been redefinitions and reclassifications of outcomes dependent on prevailing ideologies or beliefs. The question that children of all countries in all centuries have asked over the ages remains unanswered, not of biology or of the birds and the bees, but really the fundamental question is where do we all come from? Why are we here? and where are we going? This question has been asked in numerous ways and the answers are still not acceptable to all. The answer to that simple question will determine your world view or your outlook on life and how you answer fundamental questions that will define your expectations of humanity and your acceptance of the present reality. What is the present reality? A plaque of epic proportions with the iatrogenic loss of a large swath of humanity, with varying frequency and incidence depending on location of developing or developed countries numbering the thousands every minute worldwide. This is not unique to our present century as children over the centuries are recorded as the most vulnerable and endangered group, in historical records for instance, children have been sacrificed to various deities from moloch, Baal etc., state sponsored endeavors for example as recent as China's one child policy and forced abortions , India's government organized mass abortions, Uganda's Idi Amin's attempted extinction of whole tribes with children receiving the brunt of the brutality, Rwanda's Tutsi massacre , Hitler's Germanys Jewish holocaust, Herod's massacre of Hebrew babies in Jerusalem, Egyptian pharaoh's massacre of Hebrew babies in Egypt and so forth, Ultimately the great loss is humanity's which has been deprived of the great talents, treasures, and the time we will have had with them, who knows, perhaps cures for cancer, hypertension, genetic disorders and many others have been lost in this process.

How do members of the esteemed medical profession who take an oath to first do no harm, participate in these actions albeit enthusiastically and passionately under no duress and without remorse at all? It will definitely require a major redefinition of commonly acceptable norms and a process of dehumanization.

Why do the mothers of these babies participate in their terminations? That second question is perhaps easier to answer and understand, principally the responsibility lies with men. The babies originally came from men and the right environment for their nurture is dependent on same men.

Why do these things happen? Confessions of a terminator is written to illuminate or throw some light on these issues. It is written for such a time as this with believers on both sides of the divide, it is written to bring reconciliation with families and with conscience.

INTRODUCTION

The Foundations

If the foundations be destroyed, what can the righteous do? Psalm 11:3 KJV

This is a very unusual story as it may appear to be an autobiography however this is more than just that as it cuts across situations, circumstances and realities. It is initially set in the northern part but later extends to the southern part of Nigeria at a time when it was relatively peaceful. Nigeria has been in a state of flux even since the civil war between the North and South. But finally after a number of military regimes, there was finally a civilian democratically elected government and there was peace even in the midst of a restive army now in the barracks. This is of course a gross simplification but suffice it to say that there was a semblance of peace in the nation.

Now, I will have to step into the mentality of the 1980's to remember and portray this as realistically as possible.

Some names and places may have been changed to protect the identities of individuals and institutions most of which are still living or functional.

I had just finished lower six and high school finally "with most of it spent in the boarding school", and with the help of my Father applied to the University in the North East a present day hot bed in the country. University in the South was what was expected of me since I had graduated from a premier high school in Lagos however my time in boarding school had the undesirable effect of leaving me with some degree of what I now recognize as post-traumatic stress disorder, long before the terminology was coined. I had attended boarding school for the entirety of my time in the formative high school years, and had some very deep wounds that were only starting to heal in the last 2 years. Fortunately or unfortunately, it was required for all juniors and seniors to have a career day for counseling and then subsequently for the seniors, a trip or a tour of the local University. That tour suffices it to say brought back dark memories of painful moments. In summary, the premier southern university at that time reminded me of all the bullying I had endured in boarding school and it also appeared that the afore mentioned seniors were waiting for you to join the college to continue the carnage so to speak. There was also the matter of intense family dynamics between members of the family i.e. my Father and Mother, Stepmother, etc., and which influenced my choices intensely.

Choosing medicine for me as a career was a given however, based on three premises, Firstly the professions were dependent on your bent in high school towards three groups, the social sciences i.e. geography, economics and mathematics, the arts i.e. English, History and literature, or the sciences i.e. physics, Biology and chemistry, now there were supporting subjects of course and everyone had to do English and Mathematics. There were aspects of the sciences that were perceived to be more geared or directed towards certain professions, for example you may have a bent towards science but not to extreme abstract science i.e. Mathematics, additional mathematics or calculus, physics and chemistry as the base, these students tended towards engineering, teaching of the sciences, and applied sciences like geology.

There were also certain rules put in place to aid decision making, for example, even if you did well in all subjects, you still had to make choices as you were not able to do all the subjects for example, it was either English literature or Physics, History or Chemistry and so forth.

The second premise was personal experience i.e. the helplessness I felt when we lost my grandfather to probably respiratory failure and the deep down feeling that death was unnatural.

The last premise was the mentoring experience of rotating in my uncle's hospital (The Ethiope Hospital) which was a considerably large hospital at that time, it had departments of Medicine, Surgery, Obstetrics and Pediatrics, and others included Nursing and Pharmacy. It also had many inpatient beds and an outpatient department where I spent the largest amount of time. This was usually during the long vacation or summer holidays in high school.

I remember the excitement even now of observing surgical procedures and observing the art of history taking, this expanded my imagination-of the possibilities of medicine over coming limitations. This was not localized to medicine as prior to that I had spent some time in my Dads office where I was underwhelmed by the sheer boredom of running a business, balancing payments and sitting in for shareholders meetings, all important things of course, but absolutely of no interest to me, spending time with my lawyer uncles was no different. I had very little inclination to the arts and only started appreciating poetry for instance when I started dating many years after college.

This story begins in medical school Northern Nigeria West Africa.

JUNIOR, INTERMEDIATE AND SENIOR ROTATIONS.

We will jump forward by at least 3 years in medical school now, to our rotations in the dreaded obstetrics department, the obstetrics department at the University of the North was extremely busy and was responsible not only for the private and some general patients in the university but also the state owned general hospitals where we all spent revolving weekends to cover the labor ward where deliveries were fast and furious. Over 90% of these patients (in the general hospitals) had no prenatal or antenatal experience or even help. Typical evaluations that I can remember consisted of assessing the state of delivery preparedness, what was the age, how many children, previous history, medical problems, previous deliveries or surgeries, previous Caesarian sections etc. examinations-will include degree of anemia (they were almost all anemic), vital signs, cervical dilatation and most importantly the pelvic assessment. Essentially our experience in the general hospitals were mostly in high risk deliveries and sometimes the inevitable Caesarian sections due to the failed trial of labor in patients with inadequate pelvic assessments. In order to ensure accuracy, I am strictly relying on my memories of that time in the mid to late 1980's possibly 1987 during senior posting. The standard text book then was Fundamentals of Obstetrics and Gynecology by

Derek Llewelyn Jones which transformed the medical student reader to an academic specialist in a short time (or so we thought). I can also vouch without any apologies, that a few weekends amid the junior and senior postings were enough to make you either hate the craft or love it. I can easily say at that time I was among the former.

The period can be placed sometime in 1986 or 87 towards the preparations for the examinations of our intermediate clinical year of Pediatrics, pharmacology, microbiology, pathology, obstetrics and gynecology, this was way after our basic science rotations of anatomy, physiology etc. and we had survived the slaughter, which decimated at least a third of the class. We were feeling very confident especially after finishing our dermatology-rotations with the venerable Professor Dr Alabi and we were preparing for our senior postings. After our usual game of chess in the front of the male medical school hostel section, we were approached by a rather older gentleman, to us then he looked older, I guess to most 19 to 21 year olds everyone then looked old, he had with him a young appearing girl who appeared very shy. I think we all pretended not to see her, even now I cannot actually visualize her face. He asked us for a particular doctor who was suspected to be open to performing pregnancy terminations. Now we had never seen one. We realized he was actually from the North and initially were thinking this was some sort of trap. You see most of us in that group playing chess were from the middle belt or the South and abortions or terminations as we called them, were not only illegal but could get you in trouble. Now don't get me wrong, we had no clue of how to do it but we did know this student physician who at that time was a senior medical student. He was known to be very brilliant and loud and we did not want to be the instrument of his career demise.

He appealed to us for help and explained his situation, he was supposed to be the father to the girl who had been impregnated by either a rapist or friend or both, she threatened to kill herself rather than have the baby and he was looking for a place to do it safely. He had heard this doctor did these procedures and did not know what else to do.

Well, we really did not believe him, first of all, we were sure he was the father of the baby, he may also be the father of the girl, so we are talking of incest which at that time was so odious to us, and we were kind of disgusted at the thought. Then secondly we still had at the backs of our mind, a possible set up being planned possibly by the authorities.

We sent him on his way, as we were aware this particular possibly targeted student was not in the medical school hostel at that particular time anyway.

I became aware that one of the other students who came from the area of that student later informed him of the visitor. I know definitely because of the public nature of the appeal, no procedure was done for the girl.

Approximately three weeks later, while rounding in the gynecology wards, we were called to the emergency room for a young girl profusely bleeding, we all rushed there with the residents and the consultant, and lo and behold, it was the same girl again, in a very bad way, I believe she survived but barely so, and I still remember her looking at me when we got to the emergency department.

That was my first experience with a complication from an abortion. I later found out that this procedure had been carried out by a pharmacist in town who was also popular for aiding in this procedure. The man was nowhere to be found at this time.

The rest of the rotation was otherwise uneventful. However this experience remained with me a long time and became the reason why certain choices and decisions came much later. I generally excelled in those postings but never really developed an affinity for evacuations, which was the procedure to complete some incomplete natural abortions. These were very common but looked somewhat dangerous to me, also I still could remember this particular girl.

The New Life; The actual beginning

During the writing of this book, I was listening to an interview of a man who had organized an abortion for his then girlfriend and had written that all he remembered was that he paid for it, the details otherwise had escaped him, he therefore wrote a letter to the girl in question and sent a copy of the book prior to publication and asked her opinion if his memory was factual. She responded and began a long discourse, she remembered that he wanted to go to college and felt a baby would cramp his style, and he actually went on to college forgetting her, she remembered the isolation, with him not being there for her, she remembered the pain of the procedure, she remembered the loneliness and longing for the baby afterwards, she remembered going through a ceremony many years later to properly bury the never born child, she remembered way more than he knew, immediately a sort of relative amnesia lifted from me , and I remembered the real first experience of abortion, and it was nothing to do with complications from the procedure but with the actual experience of the procedure, the losing of life. Amazingly I remembered my first-ever girlfriend, we will call her name Nellie or Nell for short.

I first met Nell after the orientation week and it was kind of admiration or love at first sight at least for me, she was an accounting student, and the students in accountancy were an astute bunch and considered the social sciences apex predators, their legendary head of department was famous on being brutal, it was also mostly a male dominated enclave, so in seeing a girl there was a turn on of some sorts. it required many days and weeks of reaching out to initially know her name and then later to become friends for it to be a reality for her, she was very interesting and very focused and I needed that since I was in pre medicine at that time, she was an accountancy major student and in a very tough department. The head of accounting was famous but more than that feared by the entire university for his extremely uncompromising high standards and high expectation of every student in his faculty.

The culture shock started for us all quickly after orientation, for those of us in pre medicine, the competition was fierce as all science students were given an opportunity to excel and hence get a position in medical school. There is so much to talk about of this time, but I will focus on the events related to Nell. Our relationship was initially platonic and more than complimentary, possibly symbiotic, we were reading partners and very focused on our different subjects and hence strengthened our educational endeavors.

This continued for the first year and we did well in our respective examinations. Things started to change after we returned from our various vacations. I had spent mine doing a clinical rotation in my uncle's hospital where I did a rotation in a number of departments including the nursing, the pharmacy and the medical clinics. I had done well in my examinations however due to the academic politics, it still required the intervention of my Father to enable me secure a spot in the preclinical class. This left a pretty bad taste in the mouth but I was getting over this when Nellie told me of her vacation.

She had spent a lot of time in her father's firm and had been introduced to a guy, who was very interested in her, they went on a date, and as she later described he attempted to become physical or have his way which she resisted, and got away from him. Of course after the holidays, we both spoke about our experiences, and she attempted to reassure me of her commitment or faithfulness with minimal results, I had actually resigned myself to the expectation of splitting up and the effort to reassure me got us in a very compromising situation and one thing lead to another, before we knew it, we had crossed the threshold and got intimate to a degree that was completely unplanned, suffice it to say, a few weeks later, she informed me that she had missed her period. It is funny thinking about it now, but then there was a numb feeling that we would have to get married or something like that and it did feel right. There was a distinct lack of panic on my part but this was definitely not a mutual feeling and while I was talking about talking to our parents etc., maybe engagement, she had made arrangements with her friends and a few days later, I was informed that she was no longer eating for two so to speak. Just like that!

The medical college years

During the last two senior years, Life suddenly appeared to slow down, this was a period when there appeared nothing that could satisfy, I had somewhat excelled in studies, with a distinction here and there and well done in a few others, I had already come to the conclusions that pediatrics and gynecology were not my forte, I felt very competent in these subjects of course but could not see any real future in them, unfortunately I could also not see a lot of future in the rest. I definitely liked cardiology and vascular medicine but the limitations of the environment and society appeared to limit optimization in this area of medicine, the rest at least to me was repugnant, immunology was very interesting but it's practical applications at that time were lost to me, I like procedures but there did not appear a lot of thinking in surgery, and I am still a thinker. The home front was no better, I was at that time having to deal with a lot of disharmony with Mom and Dad with expectations completely out of whack, with a feeling of having to do a balancing act every day with each one looking out with their own selfish perspective in mind, at that time there was not only a cold war but a hot one, no communication, and abuse was rife.

We had focused on our studies in order to not have to think about these problems, it is difficult to explain a sensation of emptiness or fatherless ness in the context of a present father. My relationship with the so called religious group was no better. A bunch of Christians had witnessed to me, to the best of their ability, but unfortunately for them, they had no grasp of their material and I happened to have had a pretty good working knowledge of the subject as taught in high school and actually graduated with a distinction in what was called religious knowledge or Bible knowledge. A few simple questions which were not answered, was enough to put them off their game and nothing at that time seemed to come out of the witnessing. Their attitudes were sullen and they did not exude love or anything that I needed.

On the educational front however I felt comfortable in the now, and did not think my life was going to be any different or better if I did or did not lean to their persuasion.

Relationship wise I was also in a morass and had lost interest in relationships as a whole, I had virtually tried everything that I was prepared to try, (I had no intention of hurting myself), so I avoided bitter or painful choices, tried smoking for instance once, and never went back after almost coughing up a lung, I had actually broken up with my girlfriend Nell, then of almost three years now.

We first met in my first year in the university and we realized that we had common interests in the sense that we were both from the South, both liked hard work and both were adventurous. We dated for about two years and we're really close until her senior year. The first chink in the armor occurred during a cultural day for a lot of tribes from the south, it consisted of a large number of dances, displays, masquerades and plays, it was very interesting and each cultural group had some kind of presentation. I should not neglect to mention that this occurred during the preparations for Ramadan which was a very important religious fast for the Muslims. In retrospect, it may have been insensitive to have it so close to the beginning of Ramadan but for me, I didn't know any difference.

During the final night of the program, the main hall was attacked by a large number of masked individuals all in black and wearing turbans wielding all manner of weapons, during the scuffle, one of the Individuals attempted to stab me in the neck but due to my attempt to defend and parry him off, I instead was stabbed in the forearm which I only noticed much later with all the blood I saw on my shirt sleeves and shirt. This made me examine reality, I could have died if the assailant had his way, Now Nell, who was Muslim did not think that they had done wrong and the beginnings of a clash occurred for the first time, our arguments become very frequent and she later suggested we take a break from each other just before she graduated

The other reason for our break up was a little more sensitive and painful for me, during this relationship, she may actually have had at least 1 abortion, she never told me till after the fact and I completely was in the dark during the process. This was probably because I felt that this was a good opportunity to get married, however knowing that her dad was a staunch Muslim may have influenced her decision to not be involved with a nominal Christian. I can tell you already, my perception at the end was definitely that abortions or terminations were done without the father having any say, and l felt very helpless at these turn of events.

Suffice it to say, when she decided to leave, for a while I felt it was for the best. This was the situation when a revival meeting was started and an evangelist came into town invited by the local university scripture union hosted by the local University student Christian church.

I do not remember very-much about the meeting I attended except the heavenly sounding music which completely overwhelmed my senses, there was a call to receive Christ and I found myself standing up, I stood up and answered the call but had no idea what had happened.

One thing I knew, I was no longer the same, my old life of study, girls, books, and more girls was turned upside down, I suddenly grew a conscience and was sensitive to people's feelings, I also was unable to go back to the things I was used too. I still do not remember the name of the evangelist but that was the beginning of the new life for me.

An existence I was not going to understand for over one year.

A fish out of water

Therefore, if any man be in Christ, he is a new creature: old things are passed away; behold, all things are become new. 2 Corinthians 5:17 KJV

This became a very confusing time for me, First of all, I was infamous in the local Christian community's first of-being how to say it , too far gone, I was famous among the university community of being the hunter and always getting my prey, I had dated a number of ladies and to my shame, I could only keep track of them by ensuring I only dated ones with familiar names like Mary's etc., I also had possibly come forward for an altar call "after great encouragement" before with no change what so ever. Anyway, the end result was there was no follow up for me once the evangelist left town.

It was also a busy time as after this, I had final examinations and was actually looking * forward to possibly a distinction in Surgery, only thing I had left to do was the oral examination popularly known as the viva voce.

This turned out to be a disaster and unfortunately even though I had the highest score in the written and objective examination, a fail in the 10 points out of a 100 in the orals meant you failed the whole examination and have to retake it, this only was done for those who passed the rest of the examination, as a fail in the written and the orals meant repeating the whole year. A few colleagues and I automatically became unpaid interns and spent the entire vacation in the teaching and general hospitals working and studying for the re sit examinations. What however started out as a disappointment eventually became a blessing, my foundation in surgery and a lot of other subjects became solidified, I practically read the entire textbooks of general surgery, Medicine, tropical medicine and obstetrics.

The examinations were essentially a formality as I not only excelled in them but even other options for alternative internships opened up due to my new found notoriety.

My internship year which was done in a different university teaching hospital was very eventful for tough training but significant confidence building. It was here that I got invited to a full gospel business fellowship meeting where I began to understand the new life of a Christian, and eventually found a local Church, I also significantly improved my skills in the surgical specialists including obstetrics. This was a busy program however and my time in Church was few and far in between, this eventually left me with a passion for more of the word and love for gospel music. It was not long afterwards that I started my rotation in the mandatory one-year government program in the Rivers Delta area of Nigeria.

During this one-year compulsory paramilitary government service in the south area, I did some moon lighting with a Doctor from the Kalabafi area in a large town called Okoluko, he was extremely competent and taught me a lot, including of course induced terminations or abortions.

FIRST BLOOD

Dr Nubianoru, name again changed to protect his identity, was a doctor's doctor and a very generous man, I later realized or understood that it was beneficial for him that I was comfortable with all he did, so he could have more breaks or open extra clinics and avoid any crisis with the conscience.

The first patient reviewed again was a patient who had undergone a botched abortion from a popular pharmacist in town who secretly did abortions. She was probably in her late teens and very extremely pretty. She was rushed to our clinics in septic shock, the first hour was spent resuscitating-her with numerous gallons of fluid to no avail, she was started on pressers and antibiotics and subsequently a thorough external and internal examination including imaging revealed multiple uterine perforations, intestinal perforations and an incomplete uterine evacuation. She required resection of the damaged intestine, evacuation of the uterus and uterine repair, she was eventually to undergo multiple operations and courses of antibiotics leaving her partially deaf and probably infertile.

The irony of this situation was that despite all that she went through, she had not succeeded in terminating or getting rid of the baby, the abortionist had seemed to touch everything except the one thing he was supposed to be doing.

It was probably possible to save the baby however our use of extremely toxic and potent antibiotics will have left the baby severely deformed in terms of the visual and ocular apparatus, also in the process of repairing the uterus in context of the baby present, will have prevented adequate contraction of the uterus and therefore more bleeding, and hence we elected to complete the abortion or evacuation. We were of course not only dealing with the critical condition of the girl but also the multiple lacerations with significant bleeding and hence our focus was trying to save her life and not even if we wanted to, to save this complicated pregnancy. Looking back, terminating the pregnancy was deliberate and needful and occurred in the context of repairing the uterus and hence saving the girls life. But from then on my outlook on terminations was significantly altered, and due to significant mental and physical boredom and maybe unconsciously to escape my swirling thoughts now, of this experience and place, I volunteered for the flying doctors service , this was a paramilitary program that combined the coast guard Air Force which initially had helicopters and the national corps service, which then posted promising young graduates who had completed the paramilitary training in the teaching and medical arms and were then posted to the island villages in the underserved areas of the coast, this was at that time called the flying doctors service, it however due to corruption over time devolved to become the flying speed boat service where graduates i.e. teachers, doctors etc. were speed boated to various islands.

I volunteered and almost immediately I received a redeployment to the islands in the coastal part of the country. My initial exploratory visit was disappointing as these islands had no power for most of the week, excess energy from the off shore drilling companies was offloaded to a rudimentary power grid which overloaded and blew up the few local light bulbs once or twice weekly in one or two of the islands, there were no restaurants, or places to buy anything. There was an elementary and high school which served the three island state, also there was no longer a flying doctors

service, transportation was by speed boats and by the locals who were working for the coast guard, I did not see a single helicopter in all my time there, as I looked around, my idealism went up in a puff of exhaust smoke from the speed boats. The islands had two hospitals which were really glorified health dispensaries, the one at the sister village had a better operating room which had fallen into disrepair while my hospital was more focused on maternity care and had a maternity nurse.

I was taken around the islands on a trek that lasted over almost 2 hours because of the various stops, there was no real roads only bush paths, possibly bicycle routes, for one who could use them, I was also given the tour of the other village and the beautiful coast which was essentially an estuary or riverine coast feeding the delta to the ocean.

It was there I met my predecessor who was the main abortion provider for the region and was also supposed to be marrying a local girl from his island and moving to a permanent spot in the provincial capital. His hospital was about the same size as mine however it had an operating room-while we basically had a procedure space.

We didn't speak much but enough to know that he done well for himself. Now there were three villages on two islands and I was posted to the first island while he previously had been on the second island, I was given a house which was literally a hut, which was partially built with cement, there were three rooms, and a bed root with a bed, a small extra room and living room, there was a sort of kitchen which was very small. The house was a stone's throw from the 8 or 9 bed hospital with my only staff being the mid wife/nurse.

In the hospital, there was a small pharmacy with minimal drugs, and I immediately began to regret my hasty decision to leave my previous posting, where-I lived in the main hotel in town, had food from the cafeteria or kitchen and had my moon lighting job. Most importantly, there was no church, no radio and no constant power.

At that time however, I was optimistic that I could make a difference in this land of opportunity, there were multiple areas of need, due to no drinking water and using the river as a source of water gave rise to multiple waterborne diseases, multiparty was an epidemic and school was closed to any pregnant girl, she was also expelled from home and sent to the family and home of the boy where she became literally a slave for this family. The usual problems like malaria, typhoid, guinea worms, schistosomiasis and infections were noted, problems like diabetes mellitus with its attendant complications like leg wounds, amputations and hypertension, there were also usual problems like large incarcerated hernias, eye infections, abdominal pain from multiple problems.

I started on some basic primary care approaches like supervising the digging of wells for water, immunization for the children and some adults and sex education which was later to cause significant resistance and reaction from some aspects of the community.

The first foray into abortions was actually very straightforward, this was to complete incomplete abortions which may or may not have been spontaneous. But from there, it was called therapeutic, induced, chemical or mechanical termination.

THE MUNDANE

From then on, my life was significantly regimental, in the morning, I went to the hospital to round on any admissions and inpatients, including pregnant patients. Usually the nurse would have seen any pregnant patient and will have administer some initial medications for problems like pain, i.e. abdominal or chest pains, I did minor procedures in the hospitals and did clinics in the afternoon for any patients that needed to be seen or emergencies. These came in at any time of the day. Every Friday, I did a preoperative clinic or patients with abdominal pains, from hernias, masses, possibly appendicitis, possible obstructions, etc., all these patient were operated on Saturday with a visiting general / vascular surgeon from the teaching hospital on the mainland, actually about an hour and half from the mainland. He happened to originally be from one of the islands and after a personal appeal by me during one of his visits home and the chief of the island, had agreed to voluntarily come and help in the care of the patient from the three islands. These patient usually were discharged by me within the week, the pharmacy supplies were usually purchased once or twice a month initially by the nurse but after a disagreement by me, monthly. I learnt a lot from this physician especially in the management of emergencies and stabilization for transfer to the mainland. However very few patients desired transfer and believed that nothing good came from transportation for higher level of care to the mainland. Rightly or wrongly the outcomes were bad for multi factorial of reasons, they usually presented to us late anyway and they had almost a 2-hour trip to the teaching hospital or main general hospital with the initial 30 or 40 minutes by a very bumpy speed boat. They then had to use public transportation paid for by themselves, and ultimately go to the emergency room in the hospital, where their relatives ultimately would go home and leave them there, so they usually waited for our Friday preoperative clinic and eventually surgery the next day. We operated from morning to sundown, and had power only for 2 or so days of the week and sometimes a weekday. Outcomes were good and any patient rejected or too ill for us eventually died at home from what we gathered later. There was a general fear of traveling to the mainland for health care as typically not many returned. The medical clinics were mainly for hypertension and diabetics patients, usually for control with whatever medications we had available.

The rest of my time was spent doing terminations. The obstetrics and gynecology clinics were walk in's and did not require any identification, some of the women were registered in the prenatal clinic and classes, but most weren't, some were married but a majority were not. Considering that all prospects of basic or higher education ultimately ended with a pregnancy for majority of these girls, my threshold for provision of this service was extremely low. The money to compensate me for this service progressively reduced over the course of the year. I was sometimes compensated with food products like yams, bananas etc.

Patients were typically seen in the regular clinics and evaluated, if the complaints were pregnancy related, they underwent a full examination and pelvic assessment for those who were to be enrolled in the prenatal class, and also underwent a process for dating the age of the pregnancy, for those that elected a termination, the usual cutoff was 12 weeks or three months however I could go for up-to 5 months or just under 20 weeks if patient insisted and could afford it. For the few ones more than that, they were referred for the procedure to be done with my colleague at Okoluko. This was high risk but was more or less premature induction of labor followed by evacuation of anything remaining or left.

The procedure for termination consisted of explanation of the situation, a verbal consent, and payment for the antibiotics and a procedure date which was done in the house operating or procedure room and usually the patient came with a friend. The hospital was on the outskirts of the village and blocked the view of the doctor's home from curious on lookers, it was also not on the main road to the farms. Most people coming there could also be coming to see the nurse or the doctor in the clinics.

There was also an herbalist or naturopathic practitioner and mystic-persons whose home was near the same road, all this ensured a degree of privacy to any coming to the house.

The patient was asked to leave the money in the living room and go to the small room, the friend stayed in the living room, the patient was routinely cleaned and partially draped, the perineum was isolated with a special spatula and the cervix was grabbed with an instrument, this was then progressively dilated with dilators and then the suction curettage device was inserted and contents were extracted or sucked

out, this usually took less than 5 to 10 minutes, once emptied, the uterus immediately contracted and the procedure was over, if this did not occur, the procedure was repeated. The patient was then put on antibiotics that covered the usual flora, to my knowledge we never had an infection because the antibiotics were obtained before the procedure was done. There was no follow up unless the patient had a problem but this then required registering as a patient and in a year may have happened once or twice*

After a few months, the procedure was so refined, that the extra person was no longer needed, and no anesthesia was used for these procedures, the patients also usually were on the way to the farm and were able to actually go to the farms for normal work including harvesting etc.

Many married women also came without the knowledge of their husbands as they already had a lot of children, or didn't want anymore because they were attending the elementary and middle/high school on the island. According to the reports received from the patients, their friends and the gossip mills, I had surpassed the previous doctor in the delivery of the procedure, the recovery of the patient and the lack of complications, which really was a reflection of my personal drive to be an expect optimally of any procedure I did actively. This drive had now become a monster and made a monster of me.

After the first few months, this actually went on every day, and there were at least two or three abortions or terminations that occurred daily to my recollection. There were days of course that nothing happened but also days that there was a long waiting list. The operative procedures that were also done weekly acted "now that I think of it" as cover, for the operative equipment and drugs I kept at home, as these were taken to the other island for the surgeries that were done in the other island hospital.

Nothing was taken for granted, all the surgical equipment was kept in antiseptic liquid which was routinely changed, disposal equipment was limited and since most of the equipment if possible was reused, antibiotics were liberally used.

Over time with the money which I actually started to despise I acquired a large cache and library of movies of video tapes, and musical CDs on martial arts etc., I of course acquired a television to watch the videos, a rudimentary sound system and otherwise I am unable to explain what I used the money for. I spent money quite liberally at this time.

THE CHALLENGE

After over 4-months, like this and numerous procedures, terminations or abortions if you will, it began to become difficult, the same faces started appearing again and again, the ages of the pregnancies started getting older and older and the ages of the girls got younger and younger. I began to have questions on what I was doing, this monster that desired nothing else but to excel in anything it put its hands to do, and this driving force that was now out of control. On this particular day, the girl must have given me the wrong day of her last period and my calculation of the age of the pregnancy suggested a less than 12 week baby or fetus which was pretty routine at this time. She was one of the younger ones and was brought by an older girl, I of course examined her and felt there was a discrepancy in the size but may have been fooled due to her weight and body habitus, I was also half asleep as they came much earlier than their expected appointment probably to avoid the villagers on the way to the farms, or the snail hunters or gatherers. I had let them in the living room and kind of went back to sleep for a few more minutes. It was a weekend and couldn't have been later than 6am, which was significantly early at that time, except if you were going snail gathering, deep sea fishing or to the farms.

It didn't take very long to see that I had made a serious mistake, and addressing that error became the most complicated procedure I had done up to that time on the Island. This was an over 4 month old baby probably requiring dismemberment or induction i.e. delivery, but I was not equipped to do any of that in this room turned procedural suite.

I eventually had to sequentially dilate the cervix and piece meal disrupt and suction deliver out the supporting structures for the fetus with a modified suction catheter until I was able to deliver the whole baby as one piece with a larger suction catheter. In summary it eventually required me focusing on the sustenance of the fetus by disrupting the supply, and making conditions untenable in the womb for the growing baby and then extracting literally the whole fully formed but miniaturized baby with the largest suction catheter that I had, it required some modification which cannot be described in this account.

This was a week end to remember literally and it required over an hour to sort it all out.

Looking around at my procedural suite that day, I could certainly say that It was definitely a bloody business.

The beginning of beginnings

This little baby in a bottle I kind of kept in truth, probably as a trophy, now that I think about it. At that time however, it was to remind the girl of the choice she had made in the short term, in the long term however, it was to remind me to properly examine the patient and not believe everything I hear and overall I thought it was fascinating seeing a fully formed baby that could fit into a small sample jar. Even though my emotions and intentions were purely academic like visualizing a cadaver and I had no thoughts on the matter rightly or wrongly, However in time I began to have short sketch like dreams of this little baby, walking around the rooms, there did not appear to be an implied threat and it was actually fascinating to me but I started to think about what I was doing here.

But what could I do? The social situation had not really changed, the reasons why I started doing terminations were even more apparent, there was still rampant abuse, sexual violence, in all the numerous procedures I had done, a man accompanied the girl in only 2 occasions, no men were held accountable, even to responsibly take care of the girl or the baby, no adoptive processes were in place and the girl ends open again losing her social status, getting kicked out of school never to return and the baby in the majority grows up tainted , taunted and disadvantaged. I was particularly good at what I did but who would come after me, if any at all? Will some girls have to die first?

I had to do something to stop this out of control monster, for the first time in months, the children song, "Jesus loves the little children" came back to me, I also started seeing more of the little baby actually growing to be a walking child. It is important to note that I had not been to any church or Christian ceremony for over 9 months, but I thought I was saving the life of these girls.

An idea came to me in one of these dreams which were getting more and more vivid as the days went by. How about preventing these episodes from occurring? To approach this dilemma, I began to look at situations from a supply and demand concept. The only way I could seriously stop doing these procedures was to tackle the social evils that began them in the first place.

But how can you stop these evils, can you stop the activities of nefarious men who had no intention of doing the right thing, could you stop the encounters with these girls who may be tempted by money, love, lust or longing, how about the numerous girls or women who had large numbers of children and didn't want any more? Their husbands however did not see this concept, could not take care of the babies they already had and were ready to marry more wives though they could not afford it if these was any resistance to their lust from their wives.

We began to have post-natal clinics for the mothers which were largely organized by the nurse and was generally not effective in preventing further pregnancies.

The turnabout

I woke up one morning and it was as if a light bulb had gone off, Information is power, and knowing the truth would certainly set the girls, the women and I free. I could stop doing the procedures and make it more risky and dangerous for those who did it, there were alternatives like I did mention even in the village with the traditional practitioner, the herbalist, the witch doctor and of course the nurse. The girls could just keep on getting pregnant ensuring the girls kept on dropping out of school or I could equip the girls with the information to understand their bodies and have a significant say in the process other than to say no.

There was a large elementary, middle and high school in the village on one of the larger islands and we also had a large antenatal clinic in the hospital.

I started with the school, reaching out to the principal and head teachers and discussing the problem with them, they understood the need for something to be done. They could see the high dropout rate among the girls, the understanding then was education was one of the main ways you could improve your lot in life and this school was subsidized by the oil companies in the background, yet attendance was always a problem.

I then volunteered as an instructor for the whole school, and was assigned the subject of applied biology i.e. Family planning Methods.

This project was designed to reach the whole student population with the exception of the elementary school students.

It was decided after discussion with the principal and head teachers to have this after school so as not to interfere with normal lessons but to use the large assembly hall in order to accommodate all of the students, the lessons were to be held on Friday after the last school lessons.

After generally informing all the students and the available parents on the proposed "applied biology" health education classes including Sex education, we started having the classes after a 2-week informational period.

Altogether over 23 classes were held and the format was always initially based on biology, the anatomy of the reproductive organs were described in male and female. The focus was mainly on the normal cycle of reproduction i.e. The normal menstrual rhythm or cycle was described and the presence of windows or safe periods were discussed. The girls were engaged in the process of calculating their windows or safe periods in which an extra day or so is added to the beginning and the end, this was added to ensure complete safety from chance of pregnancy.

It must be understood that these females were a mixed bunch of unmarried, married or even divorced girls. From our informal informational outreach, there was already a push back from the husbands and even some fathers. Abstinence as a policy had a dismal failure especially the married women or girls, however if the girls were educated on a particular timing of avoidance, they were able to insist on avoiding physical contact in this window period and the men eventually would comply as long as this period is specified, understood and agreed upon.

For the unmarried or divorced girls, abstinence was always raised and most of them would listen to the lecture, but reality of the number of pregnant girls that I had seen for months now, spoke of limited success, and hence the educational outreach to avoid unnecessary and unwanted pregnancies was continued in all the female groups.

Due to significant poverty, condoms were not available or affordable due to costs or cosmetic appeal. It must be clear that this was way before the HIV/AIDS epidemic presented to the delta sub-continent area, and even though infections were present, they were very few or far in between. This approach was going to change significantly with rising incidence of HIV and problem of trafficking, terrorism and abuse, but this was to come much later in less than 5 years.

The classes were heavily attended, the assembly hall was packed full, with standing room only, a large blackboard acted as the sole audiovisual aid and notes were taken including drawings by the entire student body including non-students who had been invited by their friends. Since the classes were on Fridays after school, everyone could attend and everyone did. Some teachers also started attending after a while.

The attitude and approach was to empower the audience, to offer abstinence and to remind them of the focus on education and avoid distractions, to both girls and boys, the responsibility of optimizing their parents and their individual investment in their future was discussed, the possibility of a long term responsibility a possibility of a baby for a momentary pleasure has to be considered. For the girls, especially the married ones, to ensure they had control and understanding of their bodies, to ensure that they were aware of a safe period of engaging in physical activity as we called it and they were not victims of their physiology was emphasized.

While terminations or abortions was not discussed, the high incidence of teen pregnancy in the antenatal clinics and maternal mortality was discussed.

A little discussion of the male and female anatomy was discussed but the emphasis became on practically calculating safe or window periods for all the girls attending the classes. This was always based on 3-4 menstrual periods and for those that were irregular, an extra window period was given. This was considered a non-physical period not to be negotiated if abstinence was not possible.

These classes caused a lot of complaints from some of the older men and we started getting threats in the hospital.

Interestingly, there were absolutely no complaints that I was aware of about the abortions or terminations, and even though the number of unplanned pregnancies started drastically reducing, the complaints increased exponentially after the practical biology education classes.

THE EXODUS

The handwriting was already on the wall, the environment had become noticeably hostile, some would saw toxic, especially from the older men and some husbands of some of the women coming to the antenatal clinic, however there was still a lot of respect for the doctor and staff and a lot of appreciation for the free classes that the doctor was willing to give, especially as I also started giving preparatory classes for final school certificate examinations in mathematics and biology, which were hugely popular.

The time for the sex education classes were now very short and focused on prevention, responsibility and future goals.

On that basis, I decided to participate in some revision activities of the teaching staff for preparing the students for their final certificate examinations. These classes as previously mentioned were very popular and were a regular fixture every Friday in the school now.

The year was fast coming to an end, and I was aware that my time was running out. I actually realized that I was living off food donated to the hospital indirectly and directly to the doctor and of course, the money which was coming in from the termination procedure.

The islands also did not have any banks and the monthly stipend we received was paid almost 2 hours away to a bank at Ahoada, which was the provincial capital of the region.

I finally took some time to visit the general hospital at Ahoada to watch some operations and assist in others and also visited the local bank where I realized that I had not withdrawn any monies for over 7 months.

I actually ended up not needing to do any withdrawals at the end due to all the money that was coming in from terminations. This money was never put into my account because deep down I felt it was sort of blood money and did not want to contaminate what I looked at as legal money.

On my way back, during the speed boat ride, I spoke with some people returning back from the city markets and realized the major topic of discussion was the sex education classes and the now so called liberation of the women.

The ladies were now empowered to not only be able to choose when they could physically be active so to speak, but also were excited about their individual futures, they wanted to be more than potential mothers albeit educated ones but were also thinking of life off shore, the doctor had come from parts unknown and was actually teaching classes, they all mostly had some experience with me directly or indirectly when accompanying their friends to see me but this was different, I had become relatable and there was a growing gulf between them, me and the men. I had a particularly successful penultimate class where I was sent off though the classes were being continued and at this time, I was very comfortable with the results of these classes. There was also no replacement doctor for the next year.

This was the underlying atmosphere towards the end of my rotation and I was already making arrangements to move my things from the island, my few belongings including a few electronics were being packed up.

I made a courtesy visit to the chief or king of the villages, which I used to do at least every 2 months or so as most of the food resources donated did come from the palace.

However this meeting was different, as though he expressed gratitude and appreciation for all the projects in community intervention, the health clinic and the operations which we had brought to the villages and finally he spoke about the biology and mathematics classes he had heard about. He however felt that the sex education was a little too much and the logic of this was again explained with understanding, however he made clear there were reports of strive among the families and reports had been coming to him.

He agreed though that the cultural shift in empowering the whole young population would come with some complications, that is making an omelet would require some eggs to be broken, some cultural eggs or ceilings had to be shattered.

There was a ceremony to thank the medical staff and the doctor which was very formal and during this time, I was informed of some more planned celebrations and a plot to possibly protest the classes and the so called unintended woman's liberation, which potentially could be an opportunity for mischief. I received some more heads up that mischief or malfeasance was being planned.

After saying good bye to most of the people and taking a break of the celebrations, I made my way with a few suitcases to the beaches, this was not unusual as I had been transferring electronics etc. to the mainland, but this time, I also got on the boat, the last boat for that day and headed out of the island.

THE RECKONING

After this life became a blur, most of my activities of this time have really been forgotten, some sort of amnesia. I recall staying with some friends including seeing a girlfriend and relaying my plans to leave the state.

I started investigating opportunities for specialization, and temporarily looked for some local work while I explored the opportunities to do a specialization for optimum outcomes in a specific field, I speculated on orthopedic surgery and vascular surgery, my choice area had always been cardiology but in Nigeria there was significant limitation in the basic equipment, even twelve lead electrocardiograms were not available, and throughout my cardiology rotations, we used only single lead ECG strips which were generally 10 to 15 years behind the rest of even the developing world . Surgical procedures were therefore more attractive as differences could be seen immediately after intervention and patients could feel the differences right away. Cardiology on the other hand seemed to be about making great diagnosis but eventually the patient joined a long waiting list for referrals or died while awaiting definitive procedures or the procedures were just not available.

The limitations in specialization were also considerable because of the earlier senior exodus, this look place at two levels. First the local association of resident doctors, the senior registrars, registrars and senior house officer's association was significantly involved in advocacy for the medical profession regarding the substandard equipment available in the hospitals for their training and subsequently for the benefit of the patient, and the lack of medications. At this time medical care was free in Nigeria or substantially subsidized and the very low salaries, brought them into conflict with the military government. Eventually a strike was called by them and the military responded with a crackdown, there were arrests and a lot of these doctors especially the officers of their association left the Country. Most of them never came back and the rest of the resident physicians began to explore opportunities to leave the country also.

Now with a lot of the middle level physicians gone or going, it did not take long for the consultants and professors to start exploring other options. They may not have joined the strike largely for ethical reasons, but they were in support of the ideals or reasons for it. They understood though that direct confrontation would not work for this government and since most of them trained abroad, it was not difficult for them to start leaving also for parts unknown. This initially started as a trickle but later became a fast stream, the professors went initially to the United Kingdom, United States and Europe, but eventually the Middle East i.e. Saudi Arabia, United emirates and more. Now with this (I called it) senior exodus, even the oldest schools became emptied-of their professors and consultants, the reasons for this were downright financial unlike the altruistic reasons and causes of the resident doctors in training, these professors spoke of the large salaries and benefit packages especially when they came back yearly during the annual specialists and medical school examinations.

It did not take long for their examples to be replicated by graduating classes of medical doctors with sometimes whole classes leaving the Country after graduating, even the mandatory national youth service programs were no longer considered important and the eagerness for graduate doctors to seek opportunities for service has been completely eroded.

This was the situation when I returned from the program, large numbers of my colleagues were abroad and this was more especially pronounced in the southwest and eastern schools.

It was at this time, that there was an intense yearning and hunger for the word and presence of God and I attempted and reconnected with my faith and with Church, however, my perspective of Christianity as practiced at that time appeared to be cult like and based on larger than life figures who commanded intense devotion from followers, and I once again was reminded of why I was put off by organized religious activities.

I could still identify with the call of God, and I recognized that he had not given me any peace in the process over the months and even with what I called the empowerment program, I was the one that needed peace from the pain of these lives more than the mothers or fathers themselves. Seeing the little baby reminded me of something I read somewhere in the Bible about God fashioning all the secret parts in the dark, the dreams of the walking little baby had ceased a long time ago after I started the talks but I remembered what the Bible had said about where the babies come from and were ultimately going back to God, I knew that there will be a reckoning and accounts will someday have to be settled.

THE REAPER COMETH
(For whatsoever a man soweth, that shall he also reap)

When I finally got home there was a sense of the calm before the storm, it was difficult to explain then and only now as an afterthought can it be put in perspective. We were staying at one of our homes in a place called Festac town, this was a reasonably nice home of at least 5 or 6-rooms I think, there were two big living rooms, upstairs and downstairs, with all the posh stuff usually downstairs. Including the special China, big televisions, and expensive chairs etc. My Fathers office was upstairs, his room was next to the office and his Bedroom and bathroom were next to this room. I think there was a guest bedroom upstairs too but I am not sure. My stay in that house was very brief at the end.

Downstairs was "other than the large living room which I have already mentioned ", also the kitchen, the bathroom, including toilet or restroom as it is called in the United States, and our bedroom, which I suppose could also be a guest room. The rooms all had iron bars on the windows which were especially small.

Now our room consisted of a large bed and a bath room toilet combination. It also had all my videotapes, Albums, CD's etc., my sound system and television were also in here and a few other things including a lot of large suitcases which I brought from my sojourns in Rivers state. All my suitcases contained cloths, books and all my operative equipment were also in the rooms.

On my arrival, I was reintroduced to my cousin Ed and of course my Brother Jesse junior was home for the holidays from the University of Elafe. School of law. Ed studied English in College and was very interested in journalism, he was staying with us while his applications for a journalism job go through, Jesse was home for vacations and so we all had a reunion of some sorts, we were not to all see each other again for over twenty years but we didn't know that then.

We did a lot of talking but little real communication, a lot of the events were difficult to discuss with non-medical personnel, and the conversations were usually very exploratory, a lot more arguments than talking, usually playing defense or interference with activities with as we like to call it the old man. I got a job in one of the local clinics and was already planning on options of residency training locally or post graduate training, when I got an acceptance letter to an Orthopedic program in a specialist hospital in Owerri state. It was interesting seeing patients once again in definitely a modern setting as compared to the last year or so.

As previously mentioned, We all stayed in a very large room downstairs and on that fateful night, I woke up sometime early in the morning but noticed something unusual, I felt I was in a dream, I was standing outside my body and looking in and around, I saw a short pygmy looking individual who was squeezing through the small window and then walking around the room, the lights in the room were on and the door was open, the corridors were all illuminated and suddenly the front doors were swung wide and were then staying opened. Meanwhile, it was still pitch dark outside and I was thinking who in the world will open the front doors at this time, then I looked around and attempted to call out and shout but no sounds came out of my mouth. I looked around and I was now lying down on the bed but could not move any part of my body, my eyes were open and I couldn't say anything. Subsequently two large men came into the room and started carrying out stuff from the room, everything was being taken, the sound system, the videos, the albums, the television sets, even my clothes were taken. I still thought I was dreaming, then suddenly the men grabbed Ed by his shoulders and feet and dropped him on the ground, before I could whisper jack robins, I felt hands holding my feet and arms and I was dropped unceremoniously on the ground.

And the bed was taken out of the house.

There was an unusual strange sweet smell in the room which appeared to be getting stronger, and that was all I remembered before total blackness descended.

Much later, we put all the pieces and events together, it appeared that through a small pantry window, a hose was inserted and an anesthetic gas was released into the house. Then a small statue person, was inserted through the small window, and he was able to open all the doors including the outside doors. The thieves stole everything that

I brought from my sojourns, all of my electronics, cloths, accessories, even the bed we were sleeping on was moved to obtain items that were still in boxes, not to talk of the rest of the house, the full extent of what was taken was still being assessed by the time I left the house and moved to start my orthopedic program in the eastern part of the country. The rest of the family eventually moved to a larger house in the same model town. The house for a while stayed empty after the move but was eventually rented out for a short while and then was sold. I never went back to that house again and even the music albums, videos, CD's etc. that were stolen, I never heard them again. It was like a chapter closed in my life but thankfully no one was hurt, no one was injured or harmed, no one was kidnapped and only property was lost. I started out at Owerri with less than my internship or house job or before my rotation in Okoloku. Strangely all that was left were my text books and notes from before my time in the rural islands and also my surgical equipment for the procedures. My reuse-able suction curettage, my set of surgical dilators and other instruments. Everything else was gone and these books and instruments were eventually taken to London after my time in Owerri which was to be almost one year after these events, but that is a story for another time. They were left in storage in London and remain there until this day in the basement of our home in New Cross Gate in London.

The strange void that existed after returning from the Islands became clearer, there was a work to be done, but not the work that I was doing, and until I started it, and rested on the work done on my behalf at the cross, peace was fleeting, no matter how many successful procedures and astute medical diagnosis could fill that space. I started to talk to God about the next step forward, but I was really asking him to bless what I felt was the way already open for me. Should I leave to London? Multiple calls from my Mother to come over had started in earnest, and after an interview at the British embassy which I had long postponed due to the humbling experience of having to line up for hours in the morning to be interviewed to obtain my passport. I had all the information needed to apply for its renewal, but had come over to Nigeria on my Fathers Nigerian passport as a dependent. My prayer then was where in the United Kingdom do I go? There was no answer, or the answer was nothing! No calls, nothing, I heard absolutely not a thing, and while I was waiting I was of course working.

I had a temporary job at one of the branches of the popular Ethiope clinics, not too far from my home at Festac, mostly medical problems and basic minor surgical urgent care needs. I could have sworn my passport was either with me or still at home, however after a usual day at the clinic, I suddenly realized that the passport was no longer on my person, it had disappeared, I searched everywhere including going back home to no avail, I could not find it anywhere. I suspected a few people but deep down after sober reflection, I realized that I was relieved that I did not have to leave yet. God to me, had spoken, he had allowed the reaper come in once again, I would have to wait on him and hear him clearly as to where to go. I had started to suspect that it was not London from then on. In a few weeks I was on my way to Owerri where the adventure with medicine and God continued. The story continues……

In summary, few comments to a number of people, to the matured believers, the need for adequate follow up of all new believers, what is referred by those in Christian circles as discipleship is crucial for the optimal development of every believer or true Christian and also for your own development, you will not grow if you neglect this important role God has trusted you with. It is not a choice, it is expected by the master, that when we abide in him we bring forth fruit and that fruit must remain, only then do we expect to get our own needs met, John 15:16 KJV: Ye have not chosen me, but I have chosen you, and ordained you, that ye should go and bring forth fruit, and that your fruit should remain: that whatsoever ye shall ask of the Father in my name, he may give it you. The words of the master ring true; Go ye therefore, and teach all nations, baptizing them in the name of the Father, and of the Son, and of the Holy Ghost: [20] Teaching them to observe all things whatsoever I have commanded you: and, lo, I am with you always, even unto the end of the world. Amen. Matthew 28:19-20 KJV.

To the new or young (not in age) believers, my experience has shown me clearly that this supernatural walk of a prodigal is still supernatural, when you are in Christ, you are not the same, 2 Corinthians 5:17 KJV. Therefore if any man be in Christ, he is a new creature: old things are passed away; behold, all things are become new. You however can be changed and still be a beggar at the gates on earth like Lazarus in Jesus story or you could be like Abraham. I was changed on receiving the gift of salvation but the absence of constant sustaining spiritual food made me somewhat ineffective but amazingly God had not given up and was still in control. Other Christians can give up on you, but God will never leave you or forsake you. He that began that good work of salvation promises to complete it in Jesus name. Never give up or give in, he loves you and will sustain you, find a Bible and find a Church, read it from John, and make sure you are taught sound doctrine.

To those who do not believe yet, I will leave you with this, Jesus loves you and came to die for the whole world which includes you, he died because we are all sinners, and God is perfect perfection, his justice and righteousness cannot exist in a rebellious state which is sin personified. We know that the wages of sin are death, but the gift of God is Jesus Christ, except you are born again, you cannot have eternal life and see Gods kingdom. Romans 6:23 KJV

For the wages of sin is death; but the gift of God is eternal life through Jesus Christ our Lord. John 3:3 KJV

Jesus answered and said unto him, Verily, verily, I say unto thee, except a man be born again, he cannot see the kingdom of God.

If you confess that Jesus is Lord and believe in your heart that God the Father raised him up from the dead for our justification after he died for our sins, you are saved, say this confession and mean it, I acknowledge that I am a sinner and have done so many wrong things, I thank you Jesus for coming from Heaven and for paying for my sins and dying for me on the Cross of Calvary, you died and were buried for me and God raised you from the dead for my justification (as if I never sinned) I ask that you send your Holy Spirit to live in me and help me live for you from now on in Jesus name Amen. Romans 10:9-11, 13 KJV

That if thou shalt confess with thy mouth the Lord Jesus, and shalt believe in thine heart that God hath raised him from the dead, thou shalt be saved. [10] For with the heart man believeth unto righteousness; and with the mouth confession is made unto salvation. [11] For the scripture saith, whosoever believeth on him shall not be ashamed. [13] For whosoever shall call upon the name of the Lord shall be saved. Romans 4:25 KJV

Who was delivered for our offences, and was raised again for our justification. Mark 16:16 KJV

He that believeth and is baptized shall be saved; but he that believeth not shall be damned. If you made this confession and mean it, you are now born again, please find a NKJV or a Bible you understand and a church home, you have access to see services from Grace International Church online GIC Global – TransformingLivesgicglobal.org https://gicglobal.org but remember you need to be baptized, not to be saved but to take a step of obedience and release the power of God reserved for the obedient Christian to be effective in his work, take your bible open it and start reading from the book of John, and the Lord will continue to help you. Follow the advice, I gave all the other groups and I pray we meet this side of eternity or if not, the other. I love you and God bless you.

LESSONS FROM CONFESSIONS

The heart is deceitful above all things, and desperately wicked: who can know it? Jeremiah 17:9 KJV

Now if I didn't address your group, this chapter is for you. Let me speak with Men, the men group.

You are the original carriers of life, it usually starts with provision and so you are the hunters and seek prey, or the farmers and bring home the provision, this is possible because you visually identify the goals and are physically equipped to bring home the bacon so to speak, however you are also attracted visually and sometimes mistake women or females as prey also, you hence invariably by hunting inadvertently may propagate the human race but it is usually a broken race.

We must remember that women are not prey, some may be fragile, but are definitely not weaker, the strength of men in this case is for protection, we must remember to treat them like fine china, and knowing the enormous cost, we protect fine china with all our strength and usually those who have no idea of the cost, act like bulls in a china store breaking everything to their detriment.

So the question to men is; what have we done? We have reached out to women by emotional blackmail, forced them to lower their moralistic standard's, calling it all sorts of things, like liberation, choice or societal advancement, all to get our way, we have blurred their emotional horizons and hence sealed the deal. But what have we done? We have taken an extra step from David, he eliminated the rival man, and kept the woman and child, we have walked away from both, ignored our responsibilities so much that, the man is no longer the protagonist, in fact he is no longer in the picture. He is completely ignored, there is now a cultural dysfunctional and dystopian situation.

On one extreme, it's all about the woman's choice, women's right to choose what they want to do with their bodies, and they choose usually what the men want to do with said bodies. On the other hand, the women are ignored, their bodies are not their own, they are just vehicles or factories all for the baby or child. It's all about the child.

My experience in confessions was that over 95% of cases that came did not come with the man though he probably provided the means for the choice. Where is the man? He probably and usually is in the same crowd accusing the woman. As in the first coming of Jesus, John8:11KJV

Genesis 3: 17-19 KJV And unto Adam he said, Because thou hast hearkened unto the voice of thy wife, and hast eaten of the tree, of which I commanded thee, saying, Thou shalt not eat of it:

cursed is the ground for thy sake; in sorrow shalt thou eat of it all the days of thy life; [18] Thorns also and thistles shall it bring forth to thee; and thou shalt eat the herb of the field; [19] In the sweat of thy face shalt thou eat bread, till thou return unto the ground; for out of it wasn't thou taken: for dust thou art, and unto dust shalt thou return.

God will hold men accountable for their dereliction of duty, they are already becoming spiritually and culturally irrelevant. They are on both sides of this divide, the elephant that is not in the room. No woman will have life growing in her if it was not first given by a man, divorcing the responsibility and act of propagation from pleasure only ensures that the abuse and misuse of women is propagated and prolonged. With no responsibility for the act, the cultural safeguards that have been put in place to preserve "fine china" are hence pulled down and torn down to the eventual deterioration of the human race. This may satisfy man in the short term, but in the long run all mankind loses. What must be done? There is a need for a recall, in fact there is already a recall notice, all have sinned and fallen short of the glory of God, but there is hope, because of the everlasting never ending love of God, even in the old covenant he makes it plain. Psalm 8:4-6 KJV

What is man, that thou art mindful of him? And the son of man, that thou visits him? [5] For thou hast made him a little lower than the angels, and hast crowned him with glory and honour. [6] Thou madest him to have dominion over the works of thy hands; thou hast put all things under his fee

Men need to recognize their situation and answer the call, return back to the manufacturer, return back to God. He alone can reset the heart and bring back his original purpose for man, this purpose is found in his Son Jesus Christ. There is no need to redefine men, some, that are assertive, are now called toxic masculinity and others that over compensate, have become effeminate, ineffectual and uninspiring, like a female male. The place to be is somewhere in between, like Jesus he is the Lion and the Lamb, you don't want to be a Lion when you should be a Lamb and vice versa, gentlemen you must go to him and learn from him, he alone can help us, go back to the final paragraph of the earlier chapter and talk to him, hopefully that chapter now speaks to you.

For the women, this is all about you, understand you have an enemy, and it's not within, he is without, and Satan hates you and has always hated you since the fall of mankind. Genesis 3:15-16 KJV

And I will put enmity between thee and the woman, and between thy seed and her seed; it shall bruise thy head, and thou shalt bruise his heel. [16].

However the good news is you are loved by God, he sent his only Son to die for you to forgive your sins and to live for you so you can thrive, remember who you are.

You are a child of the King and not any man's play thing. His thoughts for you are precious. Jeremiah 29:11 KJV

For I know the thoughts that I think toward you, saith the LORD, thoughts of peace, and not of evil, to give you an expected end.

Please receive the free gift of life and live for the only one that truly loves you as you should be loved. See the last paragraph of the last chapter also and God bless you.

For the babies, youths and children, live and keep on living for God, for your Father who is in Heaven. Psalm 127:3 KJV

Lo, children are a heritage of the LORD: and the fruit of the womb is his reward.

And finally for those in authority, parents, school teachers, the government, the judges and more, I leave you a message, I agree that we cannot legislate morality but we can put in place and carry out laws that preserve and protect life and conduct. Romans 13:3-4 KJV

For rulers are not a terror to good works, but to the evil. Wilt thou then not be afraid of the power? Do that which is good, and thou shalt have praise of the same: [4] for he is the minister of God to thee for good. But if thou do that which is evil, be afraid; for he beareth not the sword in vain: for he is the minister of God, a revenger to execute wrath upon him that doeth evil.

You can make a difference or you can be an example of the difference God will make when he removes you from the scene. Be wise, seek him while he may be found, and remember your soul can be required of you in an instance, what will your legacy be? There are still many more groups that could be addressed, but this is written not to entertain but to unload burdens and provide a way out for many.

God bless you all.

www.ingramcontent.com/pod-product-compliance
Lightning Source LLC
LaVergne TN
LVHW052003060526
838201LV00059B/3807